How to Live to be 100 Years Old, but Feel Like You're 20!

How to Live to be 100 Years Old, but Feel Like You're 20!

✦

The Golden Keys To Optimal Health

Dr. Joshua Ebert
Dr. John Kosinski

iUniverse, Inc.
New York Lincoln Shanghai

How to Live to be 100 Years Old, but Feel Like You're 20!
The Golden Keys To Optimal Health

Copyright © 2007 by Joshua Ebert, John Kosinski

All rights reserved. No part of this book may be used or reproduced by any means, graphic, electronic, or mechanical, including photocopying, recording, taping or by any information storage retrieval system without the written permission of the publisher except in the case of brief quotations embodied in critical articles and reviews.

iUniverse books may be ordered through booksellers or by contacting:

iUniverse
2021 Pine Lake Road, Suite 100
Lincoln, NE 68512
www.iuniverse.com
1-800-Authors (1-800-288-4677)

Because of the dynamic nature of the Internet, any Web addresses or links contained in this book may have changed since publication and may no longer be valid.

You should not undertake any diet/exercise regimen recommended in this book before consulting your personal physician. Neither the author nor the publisher shall be responsible or liable for any loss or damage allegedly arising as a consequence of your use or application of any information or suggestions contained in this book.

ISBN: 978-0-595-43988-1 (pbk)
ISBN: 978-0-595-88309-7 (ebk)

Printed in the United States of America

We would like to dedicate this book to our beautiful wives Keri and April, our loving families, and our patients for making us better doctors and better people.

Contents

Foreword ix

Introduction xi

Golden Key #1—Understand How Your Body
    Really Works! 1

Golden Key #2—Chiropractic Care Rocks! 13

Golden Key #3—Get Up And Get Moving! 23

Golden Key #4—Fueling Your Body
    For Optimal Performance! 37

Golden Key #5—Lifestyle Choices,
    The Mindset For Success 67

Appendix A Websites 81

Appendix B The Top 11 Questions About Chiropractic 83

About The Authors 89

Foreword

Even with all the information available today, people hunger for something real. Finally, here is a book that gives you all the keys to live life to the fullest.

"How To live To Be 100 Years Old, But Feel Like You're 20" touches on all important areas that people want to improve in their life. That is the difference with this book. It is not just another self-help book. It is empowering. This book gives *YOU* all the control. Dr's Ebert and Kosinski have done a wonderful job explaining and creatively drawing all the keys you need to truly experience LIFE. Once you understand them, you gain the control to do the best for yourself.

If you are like most people still on a quest for your true potential, then read this book. Invest in this information to better your life and to blaze a direct path toward making optimal health a reality in your life. Ebert and Kosinski have done a wonderful job in this book empowering you to live a longer, happier, and more productive life.

"How To Live To Be 100 Years Old, But Feel Like You're 20" is enjoyable, inspiring, uplifting, mind changing, and the best kept secret to transform how you eat, play, think, and *LIVE*. Read this book with the intent of grasping all of the life changing concepts.

Share this book with others. Why keep these golden keys a secret? Share so everyone you know can enjoy the benefits of living life to the fullest and finding happiness through optimal health.

April Traylor, BS, DC

Introduction

What are the "key" ingredients to living a healthy life? With all of the piles of information out there on internet websites, television shows and in books and newspapers, it is tough to decide what advice you should be following on a daily basis. It can be overwhelming, I know, and that is the reason for this book. Our goal is to help you wade through the immense amount of information out there and begin to focus on a couple of key steps, the essential "pieces to the puzzle," that you need to follow consistently. By doing this on a regular basis you will bring about incredible changes in your energy level, your vitality and your overall feeling of well being.

We probably need to start off with a good definition of health before we get too far along. People have many different answers when you ask them to define health. We wholeheartedly believe that you were not put on this earth to "just get by." You are here to be extraordinary and accomplish great things. So we don't agree with people who say that health is simply not being sick or having some disease. That is like saying that being a good student is just memorizing a bunch of information and passing a test. No, a good student asks questions, thinks about the subject at hand, studies it thoroughly, and makes sure that he understands the concepts being taught so that he can formulate informed opinions. Likewise, being healthy is much more than just not being sick!

Here is how Dr. Ebert and I define health. Health is: optimal physical, social, and mental well-being, and not merely the absence of disease or infirmity. I love that definition! It says that it's not just enough to not be sick, but you need to be at optimal functioning in all aspects of your life. Can you imagine how great our world would be if everyone was functioning at this top level? Think about some day in the past when you were at the pinnacle of your "game". How much did you accomplish that day? How effortless did everything feel? Remember how good it felt to have energy oozing out of all your pores? It felt fantastic, I'm sure, because I have these days on a regular basis, and I know how unstoppable and how confident I feel. You can have this in your life also. You just need to know which areas of health to focus on.

Is it going to be easy? No, it won't be easy, but then again nothing worth having in life rarely comes easily. I can tell you, however, that it will be simple. There are just a few steps that if you follow on a consistent basis will head down the road to optimal health.

Here are a few things that you must understand to get the most out of this book. First, that education is a life long process; it is not a one time event. The information that we will present to you in the following pages is a great starting point, but by no means is all the information you will ever need to know about these subjects. You are at the "starting line" of health. Just like any great running race, you will have some ups and downs, but as long as you keep focused on your ultimate goal, the finish line, you will do just fine.

Secondly, you must know that there is no "magic pill" when it comes to health. Those that are searching for something like that are destined to become frustrated and eventually will throw in the towel and give up. You need to focus on learning about the principles in this book, and consistently and courageously implementing them on a daily basis. You may find yourself going off course often in the beginning, but don't give up. Like any skill you want to acquire, stick with it and practice, practice, practice. I promise you will get better at it!

Finally, all the principles in this book build on one another. There is a synergistic force that comes into play when you apply them together. Each one is strong by itself, but intensifies exponentionally when applied together. One affects the next, and that one affects the next, and so on. The more that you apply and the better you get at applying the principles, the more fantastic the results will be for you.

As a bonus to you, we have added web links throughout the book and also in the appendices to allow you to further explore and develop your education in the field of health.

If you are ready to take the first step on your journey toward optimal health for you and your family, then let's begin.

Yours in health,
Dr. Joshua Ebert
Dr. John Kosinski

Golden Key #1

*Understand How Your Body
Really Works!*

Look at these incredible statistics about our body:

- The heart pumps 2.5 gallons of blood per minute or 1,314,000 gallons per year.
- The lungs use about 90-gallons of pure oxygen per day.
- The energy output of the heartbeat in a 24-hour period alone is enough to raise 3 fully loaded greyhound buses off the ground.
- We take approx 9 million breaths per year.
- There are more than 600 muscles in your body. To press a barbell over your head takes 200 of them—31 in your face alone.
- Nerves transmit their signals or messages at 300 mph.
- Stomach acid (hydrochloric acid) is so strong, that one drop of it on the skin will leave a painful blister, but the stomach is left unharmed.

Impressed yet? You should be. Your body does all of these things plus thousands of others without you having to actually think about the process. Good thing too, because I have a hard enough time trying to remembering where I put my car keys, never mind remembering to tell my heart to beat 72 times a minute, 24 hrs a day, 365 days per year.

But how does it all work? What is the structure and function of your body? I will grant you, that it can be a very complex and daunting task to explain every single function that goes on inside you. So what I'm going to do here is to give you the simplified, "cliff notes" version. Unless you are entering into the medical profession, you won't need to know how all cells interact with one another, the exact mechanism that your glands use to secrete hormones, or how many sodium ions the sodium-potassium pump pushes through the cell membrane. It's vitally important however, that you have a good understanding of the overall structure and function of your body.

When you have this information at your disposal, you will be able to make better, informed decisions in regards to your health. You will be able to see the things you are doing that benefit you, and do them more often. Likewise, you will see the things that are hurting you, and do them less often. Our goal in this book is to move you along the road to optimal health!

So here goes, I'm going to summarize our more than 7,000 classroom and clinical hours in undergrad and graduate studies into just a couple of pages.

Let's start with how the body is organized. The human body consists of several levels of structural organization and they are all built upon one another. We are going to look at the largest level of organization, which is the organ system level, because that is the easiest to explain and understand. Also, the terms I will be using will be more familiar to you. Ok, so let's move on.

Your body has 11 major organ systems. Each has its own specific function(s):

1. *Integumentary system*—(skin, hair, nails and sweat glands)—its function is to regulate body temperature and to protect the body.

2. *Skeletal system*—(your bones)—its function is to protect and support the body and assist in movement.
3. *Muscular system* (skeletal muscle tissue)—its function is to move the body.
4. *Endocrine system* (all hormone producing glands)—regulates body activities through hormones.
5. *Cardiovascular system*—(Blood, heart, and blood vessels)—distributes oxygen and nutrients to cells and carries waste away from cells.
6. *Lymphatic and immune system*—(Lymph, lymph vessels, and organs containing lymphatic tissue)—helps to protect the body from disease.
7. *Respiratory system*—(lungs and passageways leading in and out of them)—supplies oxygen and eliminates carbon dioxide.
8. *Digestive system*—(gastrointestinal tract, liver, pancreas, gallbladder and stomach)—performs the breakdown of food into usable nutrients and gets rid of the rest.
9. *Urinary system*—(Kidneys, urethra, and urinary bladder)—regulates the volume and composition of the blood and eliminates waste.
10. *Reproductive system*—(Testes and ovaries)—hormones that help regulate metabolism and the ability to form a new organism.
11. *Nervous system*—(brain, spinal cord and all nerves)—regulates body activities through nerve impulses; it is the master control system of the body.

All these organ systems perform their specific function(s) and contribute overall to sustaining you as a living organism. To give you an analogy, you can think of your body as a giant corporation. In a big corporation you would see many different departments (sales, marketing, accounting, personnel, etc.) and each has a particular job it is assigned to perform. Your body works the same way as that big corporation. In fact, we will call it the "You" corporation. Each one of your organ systems is like its own department in the "You" corporation. Each one of the organ systems has a particular task(s) to perform. Most of the time the individual departments (organ systems) stick to themselves and do their own work, but other times they need to have some communication with another department to help solve a problem. We need to have all the departments working efficiently and effectively individually, while also having the ability to communicate with one another in order to have a successful company.

How does each organ system know when to do its specific job, for how long, and in what quantity? Furthermore, if one organ system needs to communicate with another to get some help, how does it do it?

Well the answer is rather simple actually.

There is one ingredient that is essential in any complex organization or company for it to run at 100% peak performance. Do you know what it is? Every great corporation needs great leadership. Michael Dell, Bill Gates, and Donald Trump are all integral parts of organizing and giving direction to their respective companies. They are the reason that Dell, Microsoft and the

Trump organization are wildly successful. They look at results and decide when and where to do more of what is working and less of what is not. They make sure that there is great communication within the company so that they can better serve their customers.

Your body, the "You" corporation is no different than the organizations I have mentioned above.

It needs powerful and effective leadership to function properly. So where is the leadership in your body? Which one of the organ systems that we mentioned is bold enough to step up and take the lead? Ding, ding, ding…. We have a winner! The Nervous System has volunteered for the job. It has taken over as the "master control system of the body." It directs and coordinates, either directly or indirectly, every activity that happens inside you. It is like the ultimate nosey boss at work, who wants to know everything that's going on in the office, and then wants to give advice on the problem solving.

So what makes up the structure of the Nervous System? The brain, spinal cord, and all of your nerves. It is the ultimate communication center of your body. Think of it like the electrical system in your house. You have a fuse box (the brain) that leads out to electrical wires (spine and nerves) that make it to electrical outlets (cells, tissues and organs) that power everything in the house.

The way it functions is that cells, tissues, and organs are doing their particular job and they relay a message along a nerve to the spinal cord. The message then travels up and along the spinal cord to the brain. The brain interprets the message and then sends instructions back along the same route. It will decide to keep doing what it's doing, to do more of what it's doing, or to do less of what it's doing. It may also send another message to a different department to ask for help with the task.

So for example, your lung starts to breathe in oxygen at a normal rate, but at that very moment an 800 lb lion starts to charge towards you. Your eyes see it and tell your brain, the brain tells the legs to start running, so you start to run, but guess what, your muscles need extra oxygen to run, so the brain sends a message to the lungs to take shorter more frequent breaths to put more oxygen into your blood stream. Now this is a simplified version of what would go on in this scenario, hundreds if not thousands of things are occurring simultaneously, but I think you get my point. It is an absolutely amazing, complicated process and it is done automatically for you every single time.

If the nervous system controls and coordinates everything that goes on inside you, it had better be working at 100% efficiency, 100% of the time. If it's working at 95% you might have small problems popping up, if it's working at 60% you might have large problems popping up, and if it's not working at all, then the only thing popping up will be daisies, because you will be dead! Just look at the actor Christopher Reeves. He had that tragic horseback riding accident where he severed his spinal cord at a specific level in his neck. What that meant was that his brain could only talk with the cells and tissues above the injury. It couldn't talk with anything below. So his heart, lungs, kidneys, pancreas, etc., eventually started to breakdown because they had no leadership, no communications system to help it out. Just before he died, virtually everything that was happening inside his body was done by machines on the outside of his body.

Now this is a tragic and extreme case, most people don't have their spinal cord damaged to that extent. What if, however there was some type of problem that wasn't that extreme, but still hampered the way that the nervous system went about doing its job? Imagine if there was some type of interference with the messages coming and going in your nervous system? What if it could only work at say 90%, or 80%, or even 70% of its capabilities? From what you just learned about how the body functions, could you see that we would start to see health problems arise? It might show itself in a variety of ways. Diabetes, cancer, high blood pressure aches and pains, or just about anything else you can think of.

Now, here is the final and most important concept you have to know about the human body. We know how the nervous system works, but what about why the nervous system works. In other words, what tells the nervous system when and why to do its job?

Well, let's think about this for a minute. What separates the human body from a machine? Both of them can perform amazing and complex tasks. When, however, was the last time you witnessed a broken down car fix itself? How about a computer that has had a hard drive crash getting itself back into working order? You've never seen this! Simply because it can't happen. Machines can do amazing things but when they break down they can't fix themselves, they need help from a human being to get up and running again.

Your body, on the other hand, is a *self healing, self regulating* organism. That makes it more fantastic then any machine ever created in the history of our planet. Think about a situation like this for instance; you get a cut on your hand. Your body sends white blood cells to that location to fight possible infection, thickens or clots the blood to stop the bleeding, and forms a scab to help protect and heal the skin. If you have a cold, your body will use its immune system to fight the virus and remove it from your system. If you twist your ankle and damage muscles and ligaments, your body will send extra blood and fluid to the area to bring extra nutrients which will cause swelling, and will stabilize it from further injury.

With all these "automatic" actions happening, it's as if there is "something" that is always looking out for our well-being. "Something" that knows what is best for us and will try to make sure every job gets done. Science and medicine have recognized this fact and have tried to define it or give it a name. They have used terms for it like the body's inner wisdom, life, Mother Nature or innate intelligence. For our purposes in this book, we will use the term *innate intelligence* because that term is how the chiropractic profession has come to describe it.

Innate intelligence is that "special something" inside you that is always striving to bring you to optimal health. It never takes a day off from its duties, and never makes a bad decision in the management of your health. It wants you to be at 100% health all the time, and will give directions to your nervous system to make sure that happens. It is the ultimate guardian angel; always with you to make sure you are protected and kept safe from harm.

So, then it would make sense to say, "that the body needs us to keep the nervous system free from interference so that our innate intelligence can express itself through it, to bring us towards optimal health." Make sure you understand this concept of an innate intelligence working in your body, because in the next chapter I will be showing you the only health care system in the world whose sole purpose is to allow full expression of your "innate intelligence" through your nervous system as a way to prevent disease.

So let's step back for a minute and summarize all that we have covered. Your body is the most incredible machine on the planet, capable of doing more work and processing than 1,000 of the worlds top computers combined. It is organized into different organ systems, with each having a specific function. One of the organ systems, the nervous system, oversees the others, to help them do their job at the right time and in the right amount. It lets them coordinate and talk with each other when they need to solve a problem. There is an innate intelligence that lives inside us, this "special something" makes sure that we get whatever we need, whenever we need it, so that we can be healthy and protected from the world. If there is interference in this process then certain functions of the body will not happen when and how they should. Eventually you will see this expressed as some type of disease.

So that is your abridged anatomy and physiology lesson. Next step is to show you the real life example of interference in your nervous system and its devastating effects on the body. After that we will follow up by explaining which health care practitioner you can see to make sure it doesn't happen to you!

Golden Key #2

Chiropractic Care Rocks!

In this chapter we are going to discuss one of the most misunderstood and under utilized forms of healthcare in the world today. <u>Chiropractic</u> care has been around since its inception in 1895, bringing to the world a different way to look at health. Its founder, D.D. Palmer understood the complexity and intelligence of the human body and was aware that for the most part, it has everything it needs within itself, and really doesn't need much help from us.

If we want to have a discussion about disease and lack of health, then we need to go back to how the body is structured. The nervous system runs the entire show on the inside. It makes sure that all the organ systems are communicating with one another and doing their job(s). The nervous system takes its orders from the innate intelligence of your body. That innate intelligence always has our best interests in mind, it wants us to survive, and wants us to be healthy. So everything it has the nervous system do is to bring this about for us.

So what's the problem? If we have this incredible innate intelligence inside us, always striving to keep us safe, and working through this magnificent nervous system, then why do we still get sick? Where is the breakdown in the system?

I can tell you that it is not at the innate intelligence level because it does not have a physical presence to it. It is something that you cannot touch or feel, and it is always perfect in both its intention and delivery of instructions to the nervous system. The problem manifests itself at the nervous system level. The nervous system is physical matter, and all physical matter is imperfect and has flaws. All physical matter has a birth and a death, and in between, has moments of working perfectly to moments of breakdown.

So how does the breakdown occur in the nervous system?

We need to go back to anatomy for a quick moment. I told you in the last chapter that the nervous system was made up of the brain, spinal cord, and all of your nerves. What I didn't mention was how it is actually set up in your body.

The nervous system is the most important organ system in your body. Our Creator in all His infinite wisdom gave it something special to make sure that it stayed safe. It was given a protective casing, bone, completely surrounding it, to protect it from harm. Your brain is completely encased in the skull. Your spinal cord is completely incased between 24 movable bones called vertebrae. Now the bones of the skull move as one large unit, there is not much movement between the individual bones. The vertebrae on the other hand, are all movable. This is because it runs straight down from the skull, through your back and down into your butt. Just imagine trying to turn, twist or bend if those vertebrae didn't move. If you have ever had a stiff neck you know what I mean.

Remember trying to turn your head when someone called your name? You had to basically turn your whole body in order to face that person because of the lack of flexibility in your neck. Now imagine trying to play a sport, drive your car, or play with your kid while having this inability to twist, turn and bend. It would be a pretty tough thing to do. So we need this freedom of movement to accomplish our activities of daily living.

A point of great importance is that with the flexibility and movement of the spine comes immense freedom. However, on the other hand it creates enormous potential for injury. Sometimes one or more of those spinal bones (vertebrae) become misaligned with one another, and don't go back to their original starting position. This causes stretching of ligaments, cartilage and muscle. Swelling and inflammation then will appear around this site of injury. This swelling or inflammation will then cause a narrowing or blocking of the "hole" or (foramen) to which the nerves exit through the vertebrae. Pressure is put on these delicate nerves by the surrounding inflamed tissue and guess what? It causes the nerve to not work properly.

The pressure either causes the nerve to send an exaggerated message (facilitation) or reduced message (inhibition) through the nervous system. Examples could be too much or too little of a hormone being secreted by a gland. Too much, or too little an amount of white blood cells being sent to an area to fight an infection. And so on. This is where the problem begins for us. Important messages traveling through your nervous system are being *interfered* with, either going to the brain or away from it. These important messages are what keep our body functioning properly; it's what makes us healthy. And you know what appears in the absence of health ... disease.

Disease is nothing more than the inability of the body to keep itself healthy. In modern medicine we are so eager to give a name to the maladies that happen to us. "You have diabetes," "you have high blood pressure," "you have the flu." The reality is that the disease isn't the culprit. The fact is that the nervous system can't communicate properly at that time, and we are seeing a breakdown in our communication and defense system. A body that would normally be able to fight off this intruder is now in a weakened state and can't defend itself.

The disease process is simply the problem being expressed at the weakest part of the body at that time. Just think about these examples for a moment. There is a member of your family who has the flu, let's say it's your daughter. Why is it that your wife also gets the flu but nothing happens to you or your other two kids? You were in the same house, used the same restroom, watched TV in the same room and therefore were exposed to the same germs. The reason is that your daughter and wife had some interference in their nervous systems that made them unable to fight off the viral invaders. This virus was able to make a home in her body because they were in a weakened state, whereas you were strong in your defense and were able to keep from getting sick. Understand that the longer the communication system (nervous system) is malfunctioning, the worse the problem(s) will be.

This is where chiropractic care comes into the picture. Our sole purpose for being in the health care field is to find these "problems" in the nervous system, and correct them as quickly as possible. We have even given this problem a special name, which is unique to our profession. We call it a *vertebral subluxation*. As I explained earlier to you, it is when one or more spinal bones lose there proper positioning with the one above or below, causing inflammation to occur, then putting pressure on delicate nerves exiting from these bones. The result is that messages can no longer move through the nervous system unimpeded, leading to communication breakdown and eventually some type of disease process.

Many things can cause these vertebral subluxations. It may be a chemical cause, like cigarette smoke, caffeine, or alcohol. It may be an emotional cause such as stress. Or it could be a physical cause such as repetitive micro trauma, a car accident or bad posture. The causes are really too many to mention here, but suffice it to say that any stress that the body can't handle, may lead to a vertebral subluxation. Until it is corrected it will be a major problem in letting your body function the way it was meant to.

The role of chiropractors is to find, analyze and correct vertebral subluxations. There are several tools that chiropractors can use to find a subluxation. They can use their hands to feel or "palpate" your spine in order to find areas of misalignment, swelling, or aberrant motion. They can use x-ray imaging to get a clear picture of what it looks like inside, and how everything is lined up, or not, as the case may be. They can use other instrumentation, such as spinal thermography, which reads heat differences throughout the spine, which will point to the area of injury. Finally, chiropractors can use observation to look for physical signs of the subluxation manifest itself, such as redness, swelling, and postural issues. All in all, the doctor uses a myriad of tools to analyze your spine and come up with the exact location of the vertebral subluxation.

Now that your chiropractor has found the problem, it's time to get rid of it. The ways that this can be done will vary greatly from doctor to doctor. This is the part of the job that is "artistic." All doctors have their own style and personality, and so that will come through in the way that they correct the vertebral subluxation. Remember, however, that all chiropractors have the same purpose, which is to remove the vertebral subluxation; they just may go about it in a different manner. It is just like the pitchers on a baseball team. If you compare their styles you will see vast differences between them. Some throw the ball over the top. Some throw sidearm, some throw fast, some slow, some throw from the right side, some from the left. It really doesn't matter though because they all have the same goal and that is to get the batter out, they just go about it differently.

In the case of chiropractors, some will use their hands; some will use an instrument. Some will have the patient seated and some will have you lying down. Some will use very light force, others will be more forceful. Just like the baseball pitchers, the exact correction method the chiropractor uses is not as important as the purpose for doing it. Like any other type of service provider that you may use, find one that resonates or has the right personality and style for you.

How often should you visit the chiropractor to have your spine checked for vertebral subluxations? If you think about it, that is kind of a loaded question. How often should you eat right? How often should you get the right amount of sleep? How often should you get the right amount of water intake during the day?

My answer would be; as often as needed to bring yourself to the level of health that you personally want to experience. If you want to be extremely healthy, do it more often and consistently then you would if you only want to be moderately healthy. It's like anything else, the more you do something that is good for you, the more benefits you will reap. For Doctor Ebert and I, we get our spine checked for vertebral subluxations at least once per week.

We understand the importance of the nervous system and its role in our health; therefore we know that we don't want to go very long without a proper functioning nervous system. If you wanted only to be moderately healthy, then you could have your spine checked once a month. The choice is yours to make. Keep the nervous system free from interference and live a vibrant healthy life, or let some disease take over and spend your time and money fighting to get back to health. Are you the type who likes to prevent the problems from happening or the type who likes to react to them after they appear?

Chiropractic care needs to be part of your health care regimen. It will dictate the effectiveness of the other key pieces to the health puzzle (diet, exercise, and lifestyle choices). Without a proper functioning nervous system you won't be able to properly digest the food that you eat. Without a proper functioning nervous system your body will not be able to reap the benefits of the exercise that you perform. Without a proper functioning nervous system you will not be able to fight off viruses, deal with stress, and make the chemicals necessary to sustain life. Your body will not be able to get the proper rest or recovery that it needs.

Are you getting the message of how important having a proper functioning nervous system is to you? I hope so, because it is the first step, and the biggest step, on your way to living the type of life that you want and deserve.

Action Step: Go to the links in appendix A. Choose a chiropractor in you area. Call today and make an appointment to have your spine checked.

Golden Key #3

Get Up And Get Moving!

> "If it weren't for the fact that the TV set and the refrigerator are so far apart, some of us wouldn't get any exercise at all."
>
> —Joey Adams

That dreaded word we all hate to hear, "exercise." Who wants to put in all the effort to do that? The reality is, however, that along with eating healthy, this is an essential part of becoming a new and healthier you. Most of us, just as with our dieting routines, put in an effort for a short period of time only to find ourselves drifting back into the old non-active lifestyle. The newspaper, radio talk shows, and television are flooded with the talk about how out of shape and over-weight Americans are becoming. For once they are right on the mark. Most of us are living non-active, sedentary lifestyles.

We have become "the world's fattest nation!" That is a terrible stigma; we are supposed to be considered "the greatest nation on earth." We have thousands of immigrants from all over the globe trying to get into our country to live the American dream, but for what? To get fat and unhealthy? Who wants that? In my opinion *we are the greatest nation on earth* and we need to step up and start being examples instead of becoming medical statistics. Most of us go from sitting in an office chair all day to sitting on the couch the rest of the evening. By the time we finish with work we are stressed out, exhausted, and hungry; the last thing on our minds is exercise.

In reality though, if you look at all the time we spend on our couch watching television, we could easily take 30 minutes from it and put it towards exercising. The truth is most people don't really understand the importance of exercise or why they even need to exercise for that matter.

Let's start with our kids. When I was in grade school, we had 3 recesses each day, one in the morning, one at lunch, and then one in the afternoon. Today, the schools have almost completely cut out recess for more academics. Why? Does this make sense to anyone? They're kids with an abundance of energy. How can a young child focus in the classroom if he or she is screaming inside for some form of energy release? My wife currently teaches first grade, and the kids only get 15 minutes per day for recess! That's insane. They are only seven years old.

God designed young kids to run, play and have fun, not sit at a desk for 7–8 hours per day. Do we really think our kids are going to be smarter if we cut out physical activity? Just the opposite, if we allow our kids to run and play and get out their built up energy, they can relax and focus even more in the classroom. It is not just the schools fault. I remember coming home after school as a kid and playing outside until dark. It didn't matter whether it was sunny, rainy, or snowy, I was always outside running around and playing with the other neighborhood kids.

Today, our society has gotten so fearful that our kids can't even play unsupervised anymore. It seems like having kid's just keeps getting harder and harder because of the society we live in. This is, however, one area that can be helped. We can supervise them. We can delegate some time everyday to get outside and start playing with our kids, instead of plopping them down along side us in front of the television. We also need to try and get them into some form of extra curricular activities. This will get them trained early in life so, when they get into adulthood they have an understanding of the importance of daily exercise and physical activity.

As adults, we really need to raise our activity level. Not only for our health, but we need to start being examples for our kids. We are working too many hours, getting too stressed, too fatigued, and not eating a healthy diet. The fact is no matter what the reason might be, we are just using them as excuses. We have become very complacent as a society. Stress, depression, fatigue, mood swings, and many other health problems are in fact all related to our sedentary lifestyle. That's right; the physical problems that we are using for excuses are actually caused by a non-active lifestyle. Again, just like our diet, there is no magic formula.

God designed our bodies to have movement throughout the day. None of us were born with scooters attached to our backsides. Our bodies need movement; we are preprogrammed internally for physical activity. Below I have listed a few of the benefits of living an active lifestyle.

Benefits of exercise

- Increased overall oxygen intake.
- Improvement in cardiovascular/cardio-respiratory function, basically increase heart and lung function.
- Lowers heart rate, allows your heart to work at an easier, healthier pace.
- Lowers blood pressure.
- Increased HDL Cholesterol (the good cholesterol).
- Reduces the amount of body fat and allows for healthier weight management.
- Improves glucose tolerance and reduced insulin resistance, decreases the chance for diabetes.
- Reduces the risk of getting heart disease.
- Lowers high cholesterol and helps to prevent it from getting high in the first place.
- Reduces the risk of developing certain cancers.
- Helps to build and maintain healthy muscles, bones, and joints.
- Reduces stress.
- Reduces depression.
- Increases the amount of energy throughout the day.
- Improves daily mood swings/attitude.
- Increases overall needed stamina throughout the day.
- Enhances personal self-esteem.

"I don't need to workout; I'm naturally thin."

For everyone out there who has been given this blessing, that's great but I have some bad news for you if you think this way. You still need regular exercise. Just because you might be thin, doesn't mean you are not at risk to the same health problems as someone who is overweight. An article found in BBC News titled, "Thin People Must Exercise Too," stated that Dr. Gary O'Donovan, exercise physiologist at Brunel University, has found "Many people, especially slim people believe that the only benefit that can be achieved from exercising is weight-loss. This is not the case. Our study suggests that slim people need to exercise as much as others in order to stay healthy and keep LDL cholesterol in check." Dr Charmaine Griffiths, spokesperson for the British Heart Foundation (BHF) said exercise was essential in maintaining a healthy heart—no matter what your body shape. We know that for some people a low fat diet can help keep their cholesterol level low, while for some their blood cholesterol stays high no matter how thin they are. "We can all take steps towards a healthier heart by eating a balanced diet and taking at least 30 minutes of moderate physical activity five times a week." For more information on this topic go to http://news.bbc.co.uk/1/hi/health/4778274.stm.

Let's Get Moving

Ok, let's get started on our journey to a new and improved active lifestyle. The best way to get started is to join a gym and get with a coach/trainer. It doesn't matter where you are at in life; most trainers can customize a workout designed specifically for you. Having a trainer or someone who will push you each and every day is very critical at the beggining stages of your new work-out routine. You need someone their to keep you motivated moving forwards towards success. If this is not possible or doesn't appeal to you for whatever reason, there are some alternatives. There are hundreds of great exercises you can do right at home. There are free workout routines all over the Internet and hundreds of exercise DVD's available in stores. I personally recommend the book titled, "Body By God", by Dr. Ben Lerner. This book has great plans and workout routines for each day of the week, all in great detail.

Benefits of Aerobic Exercise

We always hear about aerobic exercise but what exactly does that mean anyway? Aerobic basically means "with oxygen." Aerobic exercise requires oxygen, which is involved in the metabolic processes that produce energy. This is what increases your metabolic rate, which uses up your fat storage for energy. Aerobic exercise is most commonly referred to as a "cardio" workout. For example running is a "cardio" workout. We are increasing out heart and respiratory rates. This strengthens both our cardiovascular system as well as our respiratory system. Basically it means, better heart, better lungs. Without getting into numbers for ideal heart rate zones, here is the principle to a good workout. *If you're not breathing hard and sweating, you need to pick up the pace because you're not working hard enough!*

Cardio at Home

Cardio should be done, at a bear minimum 4 days per week at least 30 minutes per day. If you lead a very sedentary lifestyle you should increase your days to 5–6 days per week. Here are a few examples of cardiovascular exercises:

- Jump rope
- Jumping jacks
- Jogging/Power (fast) walking, get the whole family involved
- Cycling, also a great family activity
- Aerobics
- Treadmill, there are many different types of cardio equipment for home use.
- Turn household chores into aerobic exercise, just increase the pace.
  - mowing the lawn fast paced with push mower
  - hand washing your car
  - raking leaves
  - shoveling snow
  - cleaning the house, inside and out

Just Beginning

First and foremost you need to begin with stretching and an easy warm-up, usually some sort of mild cardio, for 3–5 minutes. This should be performed before every workout. The stationary bike or treadmill is great for this, or a brisk walk will get your body warmed up to start working out. You should start slowly with a basic cardio program along with a simple weight resistance program. I would recommend for the first few weeks to start with cardio 4–5 times a week and add weight resistance 2–3 times per week. There is an example listed below. This would include circuit like training, upper and lower body all in the same day. There are many different strength-training exercises with pictures to show you how to perform them at home or the gym found at http://www2.gsu.edu/~wwwfit/strength.html and also http://exercise.about.com. Do one exercise for about 12–14 reps (if you can do more you need to increase your weight) and then move on to the next exercise. Rest time should be very minimal, around 20 seconds.

Sunday—Rest

Monday—stretch, warm up, followed by 30 min. cardio.

Tuesday—stretch, warm up, followed by 30 min full body circuit training.

Wednesday-stretch, warm up, followed by 30-min cardio.

Thursday-stretch, warm up, followed by 20–30 min full body circuit.

Friday-stretch, warm up, followed by 30-min cardio.

Saturday—(optional) stretch, warm up, 20–30 min full body circuit.

—Work abdominal muscle on full body circuit days, always perform last.

For those with weight (fat) loss in mind, I would keep this program for at least the first 6–8 weeks or longer. As your workouts get easier, add minutes to your cardio/strengthening program. For those who are losing a significant amount of weight (fat) and need to move on to more of a muscle strengthening/toning routine, I would move on to the pre-building phase.

Pre-Building

Ok, you have now reached the next stage in our new active lifestyle, the pre-build stage. By now you should be noticing some changes in your energy level and body appearance. Some will have greater changes than others, but you need to hang in there and move forward; changes will come. At this stage you are going to start targeting muscle groups and adding cardio with the muscle training. Instead of doing all upper and lower body on one day and cardio the next. For this stage we are going to separate upper body and lower body into different days. You are also going to add 2–3 sets (same lifting exercise, 2–3 times) and only 10 reps per set. Rest time should be limited to only about 20–30 seconds.

Sunday—Rest

Monday-stretch, 3–5 min warm up, upper body strength training for 30–40 minutes also add 20–30 min of cardio at the end of the strength training.

Tuesday—stretch, 3–5 minute warm up, lower body strength training for 30–40 minutes, 15 min of cardio at end of strength training.

Wednesday—stretch, 3–5 min warm up, cardio 30 min.

Thursday—stretch, 3–5 min warm up, upper body strength training for 30–40 minutes, 15–20 min of cardio at end of strength training.

Friday—stretch, 3–5 min warm up, lower body strength training for 30–40 minutes,15 minutes of cardio at end of lower body workout.

Saturday-stretch, 3–5 min warm up, cardio 30–40 min.

—Abdominal workout should be done at least 3 times per week at the end of the workout.

When your body starts to adjust to these workouts and you want to start focusing more on muscle gain, then move on to the building stage.

Building

By now you should be seeing great changes on the outside and feeling them on the inside as well. This stage is basically for those of you who are already down to your target weight and want to focus on increased muscle strength and increased muscle gain. If you still need to loose a significant amount of weight, I would recommend that you stay in the beginning/pre build stage until the desired weight (fat) loss is achieved. I want to stress that fat loss and the numbers on the scale don't always coincide. You may be losing or have lost the desired fat weight but, by now you should have put on muscle weight which is definitely a positive. If your not sure, most local gyms are able to measure your over all body fat percentage. This will tell you exactly where you are at in your transformation.

You are now going to start targeting individual muscle groups instead of the pre-build stage where we targeted the upper body muscles and lower body muscles. One thing you need to remember is to not over do it in this stage. This is the one stage that injury is most prone because of over use and trying to lift too much weight. In this stage we are going to do 3–4 sets with only 7–8 reps per set. Rest time should be more because you don't want injury to occur due to the heavier weights. I recommend about 40–50 seconds between sets. Ok, this stage is about size and power. We are going to work on 2–3 different muscle groups each day. Cardio is still going to be a part of your daily routine but we are going to cut down the time a little and increase the time spent on weight training.

Sunday-OFF

Monday—stretch, 2–5 min warm up, chest, shoulders, and triceps. This is your heavy lifting day. You are going to do at least 3 different chest lifts, 3 shoulder and 2–3 triceps lifts. Each lift done with 3–4 sets and with 7–8 reps. End with 10–15 min of cardio and last end with abdominal workout.

Tuesday-stretch, 2–5 min warm up, biceps and back. We are going to do 4 different Biceps lifts and 4 back lifts. Again 3–4 sets each with 7–8 reps. You should add in a few lifts to isolate forearms. End with 15 min cardio and abs workout.

Wednesday—stretch, 2–5 min warm up, full leg workout. You are going to do 3 different hamstring lifts, 3 quadriceps lifts, and 3 calf lifts. End with 15-min cardio workout.

Thursday—same workout as Monday

Friday—same workout as Tuesday

Saturday—30–40 min cardio only

Sunday-OFF

Monday—Start with Wednesdays workout (Legs), this is also going to be this weeks Thursday workout. The 3rd Monday, start with the biceps/back workout and continue to repeat this cycle week after week.

—If you want to maintain the high cardio workouts, make sure you do cardio at the end of the weight training and add minutes as you feel comfortable.

Repeat this same cycle of workouts and you will get stronger and bigger proportionally throughout your body. If you get overly fatigued, don't push yourself too hard. Take an extra day off during the week if you need the break. You don't want to wear down your body or injure a muscle.

Well, I wish you well on your newfound active lifestyle. This chapter was intended to give you an overview of the importance of exercise and to point you in the right direction. The links I included will provide you with the tools to perform the exercises and lifts described in the previous paragraphs. This chapter along with diet is something I am personally very passionate about. It seems like both of these lifestyle attributes are not being properly utilized and are playing a big part in the destruction in the health of our society. Lack of exercise and poor diet is causing thousands of unwanted diseases and even deaths every year. We can turn this huge negative into an even bigger positive. All it takes is a little motivation to get up and as the Nike slogan says, *"Just Do It."*

Golden Key #4

*Fueling Your Body
For Optimal Performance!*

> "People are so worried about what they eat between Christmas and New Year, but they really should be worried about what they eat between the New Year and Christmas."
>
> —Author Unknown

Diet is the most talked about health subject in today's society. Diet plays a tremendous role on how we feel, look, and how our bodies perform on a day-to-day basis. Today one of the biggest plagues affecting Mom, Dad, and even the kids, is obesity. Obesity is running rampant all over the world but more specifically in the United States. This problem is taking the lives of our loved ones everyday. According to the Center of Disease Control, 300,000 people die annually from obesity related health problems. Approximately 57% of adults in America are considered overweight. Granted, there are some genuine genetic problems such as hormone imbalances that aid in weight gain but these are rare and can be easily tested for by your medical doctor. Here are some of the most common health related risks associated with obesity:

- Heart Disease
- Stroke
- Diabetes type II
- Certain cancers
- Fatty liver disease
- Gall bladder disease

- Respiratory problems
- Depression

Ok, enough with the diseases let's get to the root of the problem. In today's fast paced world where both parents work, time is of the essence. The temptation of fast food calls out to us from every street corner in America. Fast food has become the quick answer to often in our daily routine to fill those empty holes in our stomachs.

But wait, aren't most of the fast food chains offering healthier alternatives now, such as a salads and even fruit. They are, but are these really healthy alternatives? If you are getting a pre-made salad or fruit bowl, more than likely there is some sort of preservative or even added sugar on these foods. Worse yet, there are certain kinds of salad dressings that actually have the same fat content as that burger you just passed up at the drive-thru. I am not in anyway putting blame on fast food companies. Personally, I can't stand it when I here about a company getting sued for giving someone health problems. The companies don't really "give" people "health problems." Their food contributes to the problem by selling an unhealthy product at a cheap price, but the individual who purchased the food is ultimately to blame. We all make a personal choice when it comes to where and what we eat.

I'm sure we don't just eat fast food all day, well most of us don't anyway. Most of us do go grocery shopping. Here is another area that is detrimental in our food selection. A lot of the food that we think is healthy is actually packed full of additives. The most common additives are different types of preservatives, flavor enhancers (MSG), and artificial sweeteners. Let's first take a brief look at MSG.

Monosodium Glutamate

MSG or Monosodium Glutamate is a man made chemical used on foods to enhance flavor. This chemical can be found in both restaurants and your groceries you bring home every week. I was completely surprised when I started really investigating the amount of foods that contained this chemical. It is found in a lot of prepackaged foods such as: soups, crackers, most diet foods, potato chips, protein bars, processed meats, salad dressings and I'm sure many more. Well, if MSG is in all these foods it must be ok, right? Well, I will leave that decision up to you. There have been a multitude of independent research studies done on MSG. Health Dangers.com reads "Monosodium Glutamate or MSG is a man-made flavor enhancer. It is now recognized by many in the medical profession as an excitotoxin—a type of drug which damages brain cells." Please visit the web address for more detailed information at: http://www.healthdangers.com/drugs/MSG/index.htm. Also, another great website to visit with pretty much everything you would want to know about MSG is found at: http://www.msgtruth.org/related.htm. Here are some of the bodily functions MSG has been shown to negatively affect:

- Brain
- Lungs

- Endocrine system
- Vision
- Hypothalamus
- Thyroid
- Pancreas
- Nervous system

Artificial Sweeteners, Not so Sweet!

Artificial sweeteners, here is another man made chemical that is and has been added to pre packaged foods and flavored drinks. It seems like these artificial sweeteners are found in just about everything these days. I'll reference a few of the most popular. The first one is called Aspartame. This artificial sweetener has shown in research studies to be metabolized or broken down inside our bodies into formaldehyde. Formaldehyde is known to cause damage to the nervous system, the immune system and has been shown to cause lasting genetic damage on a long term, low-level exposure. I could write on and on about the many studies that have been done, but instead I will again, direct you to a great website at:
http://www.holisticmed.com/aspartame/summary.html.

Splenda is the new rage in sweeteners today. Studies have shown that Splenda has caused up to 40% shrinkage of the thymus gland, which is the foundation of the immune system. It has caused swelling of both the liver and kidneys, and calcification of the kidneys. For more on this topic I suggest going to http://splendaexposed.com.

My suggestion is keep away from these sweeteners. Why take a chance of possibly creating a preventable health problem? I know there are many people who cannot have sugar for one reason or another; there are a few alternatives. There are two sugar substitutes that are all-natural products. The first one is derived from the Stevia plant. It is called, you guessed it, Stevia. This is a natural herb that has been used for centuries. Stevia was extracted and developed as a sweetener in Japan, and makes up about 47% of their sweetener market. This product is only sold in the United States as a dietary substitute, but you can buy larger quantities on the internet. Click on the link for more information about this product, http://stevia.com. The second natural sweetener is called Xylitol. This is also a natural product found in many fruits, berries, mushrooms, lettuce, hardwoods, and corncobs. This product has actually shown to have positive effects in fighting tooth decay. This is a great substitute for sugar and other artificial sweeteners. They already have products such as gum and candies with this sweetener.

I have found a great company called www.worldhealthdepot.com that sells vitamins and supplements. If you are someone who likes to chew gum they have a variety of different flavors at a cheap price. I recommend the site www.xylitol.org for detailed information about Xylitol. Just like any product, these should be used in moderation.

There is no magic formula. Take a little time and *read what you are buying.*

We really need to take personal responsibility on this subject. After all, food is the fuel that we run on daily. Have you ever put bad (watered down) gas into your car? If you have, you probably noticed that something just wasn't right. It acted sluggish on acceleration which led to decreased engine performance. Our bodies are the same way. If we eat food that is "nutritious" but, loses those healthful properties when it is "watered down" with preservatives and other additives for color and taste than we react in the same manner. Our output is sluggish and our engine does not run to full capacity.

Golden Rule to Healthy Eating

What I am about to give you is the secret to healthy eating and properly fueling your body from day to day. Are you ready? Here it is the most simple, basic concept you will ever come across. *"God made good, man made bad."* Berries, nuts, vegetables, meats, and dairy, are all essentials to maintaining a healthy body. God has provided us with these essential foods for thousands of years. God gave us these whole foods for a reason. Why do we think we can create something better by adding chemicals and toxins to our food? We have stripped away as many nutrients as possible with all the refined and processed food. Why you might ask? It is very simple—for looks and taste. Consumers want to buy the better looking and better tasting food.

So, be proactive read the labels and buy organic when at all possible.

Stop Dieting

> "I have gained and lost the same 10 pounds so many times over and over again my cellulite must have déjà vu."
>
> —Jane Wagner

STOP the yo-yo dieting. Anyone who has been on a diet has gone through this at one time or another. We make a commitment to get in shape and lose some weight. We lose a few pounds and we're feeling pretty good. All of the sudden that loss just turned right back around into a weight gain; sometimes even greater then when we started the diet.

Here is basically what happens: our body stores up fat that is not burned off into fat cells. These fat cells continue to accumulate until we start burning off the same or more calories than are taken into our bodies. This is when we start losing the weight, usually with a combination of a healthy diet and exercise program. When the weight starts coming off we are in turn increasing our metabolism, which is basically using the stored fat for energy.

As we are dieting, fat is being burned off for energy, but the cells remain, begging to be filled again. That is why it is so easy to put back on the weight that was lost. Let's say for example that we have been dieting for a few months and sure enough we start to cheat a little on our diet and then on our exercise and before you know it all has come to a complete halt. The weight that was once lost is now back and usually even a few pounds more than when we started.

This causes havoc on our bodies. Studies have shown that extreme yo-yo dieting may have a lasting negative impact on our immune function. Did you know that you could actually slow down your metabolism when dieting, for the simple fact that most diets require you to eat very little? Your body can go into starvation mode, which means it will slow down to conserve the stored energy it already contains. This is why most diets don't work.

The best diet is to not diet at all. What? That's right, you should eat about 5–6 small to moderate meals each day. This will keep your metabolism running up to speed and give you mental alertness and energy throughout the day. Remember the rule from earlier, "God made good, man made bad". You need a balance of fruits, whole grains, and proteins everyday, all in moderation. For a more in depth look at this concept I suggest the book titled *"Body by God"* by, Dr. Ben Lerner. This book can be found at http://www.thebodybygod.com/.

Fuel for your body

Water

"You need to drink more water." I know we have all heard this many times. But why? I want to really explain the reason we need daily water intake.

Water is in every tissue, cell, and organ of your body. Here is a list of the functions of water.

- Water is the substance of life. Life cannot exist without water. We must constantly be adding fresh water to our body in order to keep it properly hydrated.
- The body is comprised of over 70% water. We must maintain this amount for proper body function. Water, along with proper food, is the most important thing we can put inside our bodies.
- The body's primary source for water is the intake of water itself. Soft drinks and alcohol take water from the body. Any substance with caffeine will pull water from the cells and cause increased urination. However, caffeine has little effect if consumed in moderation.
- Water is essential for proper digestion, nutrient absorption and chemical reactions.
- Water is essential for proper circulation in the body, and flexibility of the blood vessels.
- Water helps remove the garbage in our bodies, in particular from the digestive tract.
- Water regulates your body's temperature, just as water in your radiator regulates your car's temperature.
- Consistent failure to drink enough water will eventually lead to chronic dehydration. This causes the cells in your body to become weakened and vulnerable to disease. It weakens the body's overall immune system and leads to chemical, nutritional and pH imbalances.

- How much water do we need? A good estimate is to take your body weight and divide it by half that will give you the amount of ounces you need per day. For example a 200 pound person would need about 100 ounces of water per day. That equals about 9–10 cups of water per day. A large drinking glass is roughly around 1&½ to 2 cups.

Protein

Protein provides the framework for our bodies. Protein is made up of building blocks called amino acids. Our body has both non-essential and essential amino acids. Essential amino acids are what our body requires from outside sources such as meats, eggs, and milk. Protein is needed to repair and build new cells, tissues, and organs throughout our entire body. Most Americans get ample amounts of protein in their diets. We need about 15–20% of our daily calorie intake to be proteins. That is about 1 & ½–2, 4 ounce grilled chicken breast per day. Chicken, lean beef, turkey breast, and salmon are some good sources of essential protein. If meat is not a part of your diet, there are many other natural, God made foods that contain ample amounts of protein. One main source is found in soy. For more information on meatless protein go to, http://www.vegsoc.org/.

Carbohydrates

Without going into a long, boring description, carbohydrates (sugars), are what our body uses for energy. There are two types, simple and complex.

<u>Simple</u>—your body breaks this type of carb down very fast, the "sugar high" you get from eating cakes, and candies. The all natural recommended form is found in fruits.

<u>Complex</u>—your body takes its time with these sugars and uses them for times such as exercise when you need an increased amount of energy for a long period of time. These include whole grain cereals, whole grain breads, and whole grain pastas.

Foods for life, what every kitchen needs

Chicken

Along with protein, chicken contains selenium, a trace element that helps protect muscles from the free-radical damage that can occur during exercise, and niacin, a B vitamin that helps regulate fat burning.

Salmon

Another great source of protein, salmon is one of the best food sources of omega-3 fats. These essential fats help balance the body's inflammation response, a bodily function that when disturbed appears to be linked to many diseases including asthma.

Whole grains (breads and cereals)

Whole grain foods contain B-vitamins and other important nutrients. Whole-grain eaters also have a 38 percent lower risk of suffering from metabolic syndrome, which is characterized by belly fat, low levels of the good cholesterol, and high blood sugar levels.

Canned Black Beans

Black beans contain protein, fiber, and foliate, a B-vitamin important in heart health and circulation. Black beans also contain anti-oxidants that help clean up free radicals in our bodies that can cause cellular damage.

Sweet potatoes

Sweet potatoes are high in beta-carotene. They are also high in vitamin C and a good source of fiber, vitamin B-6 and potassium.

Carrots

Carrots are packed full of nutrients. They contain Vitamin A, B, C, D, E, K, calcium, phosphorous, sodium, and trace minerals.

Spinach

Spinach is high in vitamin A, a good source of calcium, foliate, iron, magnesium, riboflavin and vitamins B-6 and C. This vegetable may also increase the activity of your immune system.

Wheat Germ

Wheat Germ is found in the wheat seed. This is a good source of thiamin, foliate, magnesium, phosphorus, iron and zinc. Sprinkle over cereals, yogurt and salads.

Tomatoes

Tomatoes are a good source of lycopene. This is an anti-oxidant that may reduce the risk of heart disease and some cancers.

Blueberries

They contain an antioxidant and phytonutrient, which improves cellular damage and helps clean up free radicals.

Almonds

Almonds contain a variety of nutrients. They contain fiber, riboflavin, magnesium, iron, calcium and vitamin E, a natural antioxidant. Almonds contain a good fat called monounsaturated. This can help to lower cholesterol levels.

Broccoli

This vegetable is also packed with a variety of nutrients. Broccoli contains calcium, potassium, foliate and fiber, antioxidants and vitamin C. Broccoli contains phytonutrients—compounds that may help prevent diabetes, heart disease and some cancers.

Low fat yogurt

Low fat yogurt contains a good supply of proteins and calcium. Yogurt also contains live cultures that provide the healthy bacteria your digestive tract needs to function optimally.

Apples

Apples are a good source of pectin. Pectin is a fiber that can have the effects of lowering cholesterol and glucose levels. They contain a good source of vitamin C, an antioxidant that aids in the absorption of iron and foliate.

Dark Chocolate

That's right all you chocolate lovers. The dark chocolate actually contains antioxidants called flavonols, which boost your heart health. Studies have shown that dark chocolate actually helps lower your blood pressure and cholesterol levels. I would suggest eating very moderately, keep track of the calories, they add up fast.

10 common Natural Herbal remedies

1. <u>Cayenne</u>
Uses: digestion, heart health, pain, skin conditions, boost Immunity
Effects: very hot
* <u>Garlic</u> also used for heart health, and possibly lowering cholesterol.

2. Wild Yam

Uses: inflammation, muscle spasms

3. Kava Kava

Uses: sedative, muscle relaxer, reduce stress/anxiety
Effects: relaxed state

4. Saw Palmetto

Uses: primarily to promote prostate health
Effects: headaches/stomach pains

5. Milk Thistle

Uses: promotes liver health

6. Tea Tree

Uses: anti-bacterial

7. Arnica

Uses: topical: heals bruises, muscle & soft tissue pain
Effects: stimulates WBCs & blood circulation

8. Cedar Berries

Uses: coughs, fevers, TB, Diabetes
Effects: promotes menstruation, decreases need for insulin, an expectorant

9. <u>Orange Peel Extract</u>
Uses: GERD, Heartburn, Acid Reflux, Indigestion
Effects: will cause burning symptoms for people with stomach ulcers

10. <u>Rose Hips</u>
Uses: increased immune function, cardiovascular
Effects: high dosages may cause bladder and kidney stones

Juicing your way to health

Juicing is one of the best and fastest ways to get all your required fruits and vegetables at one time. Did you know that heat actually destroys micronutrients found in vegetables? So, cooking them actually takes away some of the positive benefits. On average you need about 7–9 servings per day. Natural fruit and vegetable juicing is the best way to get most of or all your nutrients for the entire day in a single glass. The juice contains all the beneficial nutrients that promote healing, give you energy and help your body fight against diseases. There are actually a variety of different juicing combinations that taste great and enhance your health at the same time. For a greater understanding I would encourage you to check out this site, <u>http://www.mercola.com/nutritionplan/juicing.htm</u>.

I also suggest the book titled, "Juicing For Life," by Cherie Calbom and Maureen Keane. Their book is full of great information on all the health benefits you can obtain from juicing. It also contains many recipes specifically to help with different diseases and ailments.

My parents started juicing when I was very young, and I am still at it today. I personally own the Juice Man Junior; I love this juicer, and it is very easy to use. I would also recommend the Jack Lalanne Power Juicer; you can find this at http://www.powerjuicer.com. This juicer is very affordable and allows you to juice whole vegetables. Below I want to give you a sample of a few juicing recipes. Similar recipes can be found on the web site, http://www.healingdaily.com/juicing-for-health/juicing-recipes.htm.

Carrot Juice

Use 3–4 carrots and 2 apples.
Carrot juice has a multitude of vitamins. It has pro-vitamin A; vitamins B,C,D,E, and K, phosphorus, calcium, sodium, and trace minerals. This juice benefits bones, teeth, skin, hair, nails.

Sunrise shake

1 orange
2 apples
1 small banana
1 carrot

Tropical Smoothie

2 kiwi
1 banana
1 orange
1 mango fruit

It's So Good Shake

3 Carrots
2 Apple
1 orange

Popeye's favorite

3–4 Handfuls Spinach
1 apple
1 Cucumber
2 Carrots

—All fruit should be peeled and cleaned before juicing when necessary—

Recipes

I have provided a few easy and healthy food recipes. This will start you off in the right direction towards a new healthier you. There are many free recipes similar to the ones below found on the web site, http://www.bodyforlife.com. I recommend this site and also the book titled, "Eating for Life," by Bill Phillips.

However, there are some recipes that require sugar substitute, again I would recommend using Stevia or Xylitol.

Breakfast

Shake on the go

1 serving, on the go

¼ cup skim milk
¼ cup fat free plain yogurt
¼ cup cottage cheese
handful of mix berries or fruit of your choice

Mix everything together in a blender for a great start to your day.

Sweet Potato Bake with Power

2 servings, weekend or day off

8–10—Egg Whites
1—Whole Egg
1—6–8oz Sweet Potato
1–2 cups spinach leaves
¼ cup chopped onions
¼ cup chopped bell pepper (red or green)
2 tbsp fat free parmesan cheese
1 tsp tomato/basil
½ cup seasoned bread crumbs

Coat or crease a baking pan (sheet) with cooking spray. Grate the sweet potato into a mixing bowl. Add the remaining ingredients and mix together. Let everything sit for 5 minutes. Put everything in pan and Bake at 400 degrees for 20–25 minutes or until solid. With about 5 min. left to cook, spray some fat free cooking spray on top and change the oven to broil for about 3–5 minutes to brown the top.

Oatmeal Delight

1 serving, on the go

⅓ cup oatmeal (uncooked)
¼ tsp. cinnamon
¼ tsp. baking powder
1–2 tbsp stevia or xylitol
2 tbsp. skim milk

Preheat oven to 300 degrees. Mix everything together. Spread onto greased cookie sheet. Cook 7–10 mins.

Power with a kick

2 servings, weekend or day off

2 small-medium baked potatoes
1 8 oz. carton egg-beaters
2 slices whole-wheat bread
2 slices turkey chop into small pieces
½ cup your choice of salsa

Make potatoes into hash browns with a grater. Cook in frying pan until brown. Add egg-beaters. Once egg-beaters start to become firm, mix in all other ingredients except salsa. Continue cooking and mixing well. Add salsa and continue to mix over heat. When the salsa has thickened up the meal should be ready!

Between Meals

Power Packed Berry Shake

2 servings

½ cup cranberry juice (check label for added sugar)
½ cup skim milk
½ cup mixed berries (frozen is fine)
½ cup low fat cottage cheese
1 tbsp of organic honey
add ice cubes for desired thickness

Blend all ingredients together until smooth texture.

Fruit Salad

2 servings

½ cup low fat cottage cheese
½ cup fruit cocktail
½ cup crushed pineapple (drain well)
½ cup mandarin oranges
a few chopped almonds or walnuts

Mix all ingredients and chill. Ready when you are.

Imitation Rice Pudding

1 serving

½–¾ cup fat-free cottage cheese
¾ tsp cream cheese (light)
Dash cinnamon
Dash vanilla
4–5 strawberries sliced up
1 small banana sliced up

Mix up the cheese's, vanilla and cinnamon in a blender. Add fruit on the side. Chill

Power Snack

1 cup fat free cottage cheese
½ cup fat free yogurt
1 cup fruit of your choice
Mix all together in a bowl

Sweet Apple Snack

1–2 serving

1–2 apples
½ cup of low-fat cottage cheese
¼ tsp cinnamon
Hand full of almonds
1–2 tsp of maple syrup

Cut out the middle of one apple so that there will be enough space to put a few spoons of cottage cheese. Bake apple in oven for 5 minutes on 350 degrees or until apple is soft. Let the apple cool for a few minutes and then mix all other ingredients into the middle of the apple. Put maple syrup on the top. A healthy fantastic snack.

Lunch and or Dinner

Chicken Pizza on hoagie

1–2 serving

1 whole wheat hoagie roll
1 cup chopped cooked chicken pieces
1 cup Tomato sauce or pizza sauce
1 tsp minced garlic
½ cup grated cheese
½ cup mushrooms

Cut 1 whole wheat hoagie roll in half. Spread tomato sauce evenly over both sides. Cook chopped chicken pieces in pan with garlic and mushrooms. Spread over hoagie halves evenly. Sprinkle grated cheese on top. Put in conventional oven on 350 degrees for 3–5 minutes or until toasted. Let cool and eat!!

Quick Serve Southwest Chicken

1 serving

1 6–8 oz lean chicken breast
½ cup of chopped mushrooms
½ cup of chopped bell peppers
½ cup of chopped onions

Grill all ingredients together until chicken is cooked. Let cool and eat

Chicken Tortilla

1 serving

1 whole wheat tortilla
2 tbsp. fat-free salsa
1 oz. fat-free cheese
1 grilled chicken breast

Mix cooked chicken chunks with salsa into a pan and cook until hot. Warm up the tortilla in oven or microwave. Put chicken and salsa on tortilla and sprinkle cheese on top. Fold tortilla in half and your ready to eat

Hawaiian Pizza

1 serving

1 whole-wheat hoagie bun
1 tbsp of tomato or pizza sauce
1 tbsp of fat-free Ranch dressing, (Newmans)
2 slices of lean ham (deli ham is good to use)
1 tbsp of grated cheese
1 tbsp pineapple chunks

Layer hoagie with ingredients and place in conventional oven. 350 degrees for 3–5 min or until toasted. Let cool and eat

Chicken Stir-Fry

2 servings

2–6 oz chicken breasts
2 cups frozen stir fry vegetable mix
1 cup of brown rice
⅓ soy or teriyaki sauce

First start cooking rice, best to use a rice cooker.
Cut chicken pieces into small chunks. Cook chicken in sauce pan with non fat cooking spray until chicken is cooked. Pour in vegetable mix and cook until vegetables are soft. Pour on teriyaki sauce and cook for a few minutes.

Pour all ingredients over rice on your plate. Let cool and your ready to eat.

Chicken Parmesan

1 Serving

1 chicken breast
1 cup of whole wheat pasta
1 cup of tomato sauce
1 cup of bread crumbs
3 tbsp of parmesan cheese

Cook whole chicken breast in pan. Boil pasta until soft. Roll cooked chicken in the bread crumbs. Place cooked pasta on a plate. Place chicken over pasta and place cheese on top of chicken. Pour sauce over chicken and pasta. Heat up in the microwave until the cheese has melted. Place a paper towel over your plate to avoid spills from the sauce. Now you're ready to eat!

Chicken Soup

6 servings

2 cups chopped up chicken
2 chopped up celery stalks
2 chopped up carrots
1 medium onion
2 cloves garlic
4 cans chicken broth (low sodium)
1 cup whole wheat rotini pasta
1 cup of peas
1 tsp of parsley
¼ tsp of pepper

Cook chicken first. Add all ingredients into pot of chicken broth. Heat the soup until boiling starts. Cook until pasta and vegetables are soft. Let cool, then eat.

Chicken without the Dumplings

4 servings

1 lb. chicken breast
1 bag frozen stew vegetables
1 envelope of chicken gravy
1 cup milk
1 & ¾ cup water

Salt and pepper to taste
Optional—dash marjoram, basil, and garlic power

Boil chicken breast until no longer pink. Pull chicken apart with fork. In a sauce pan mix chicken, water, milk, gravy mix, and frozen vegetables. Bring to a boil. Reduce heat and let simmer for 5–10 minutes.

Dessert

Not really Cheesecake

1 serving

1 cup of low fat cottage cheese
½ cup ALL-Bran cereal
1 & ½ tbsp of your chose of fruit

Mix all together and enjoy

Apple and Blueberry pie

2 servings

1–2 cups apples peeled and cut into small chunks
¼ cup of blueberries
½ cup of low fat graham cracker crumbs
¼ tsp cinnamon and dash of nutmeg
1 tsp margarine melted

Place apples across a flat cookie sheet. Sprinkle the blueberries on top. Mix all other ingredients into a mixing bowl. Pour everything over the blue berries and apples. Place in oven at 350 degrees for 20–30 min. Let cool and time to eat!

Baked Apple

1 serving

2 apples peeled
1 cup cottage cheese
1 tbsp cinnamon
2 tbsp brown sugar

Chop all peeled apples into small chunks. Mix all ingredients together in mixing bowl. Spread everything over a non fat cooking sprayed cookie sheet. Cook in oven for 15–20 min at 350 degrees. Let cool and serve

Fruit Smoothie

1 serving

1 cup your choice of fruit
1 cup fat free vanilla yogurt
1 cup skim milk

Mix in Blender until smooth texture. Drink up!

Well, I hope by now you have a better understanding of what exactly *diet* means. Remember there is no magic formula or pill that is going to get you healthy. If you follow the basic outline of this chapter and the links provided, there should be no reason not to get on the "healthy lifestyle train" and change your ideas of eating for the positive. Don't get overwhelmed; take this new found way of eating one step at a time and one day at a time. Just remember two basic principles, the first being to stop the dieting and start eating the right way, the healthy way. Secondly, and most important, don't forget the golden rule for eating healthy, "God made good, man made bad." You can't go wrong!

Golden Key #5

*Lifestyle Choices,
The Mindset For Success*

> Life is a grindstone. Whether it grinds us down or polishes us up depends on us.
>
> —Thomas L. Holdcroft

> Nobody gets to live life backward. Look ahead, that is where your future lies.
>
> —Ann Landers

> And in the end, it's not the years in your life that count. It's the life in your years.
>
> —Abraham Lincoln

Amongst the three other aspects in this book, Chiropractic care, diet, and exercise, lifestyle must be addressed first. Then why did we put this chapter last? Very simple, it is *the golden key to having success* in all the other keys that fit out healthy life puzzle. If you start off your new way of life with the same habits, same bad attitude, and the same stressed out lifestyle then you will not be able to achieve the positive attributes that come from each one of the previous mentioned keys. The way we live our lives, view ourselves and others, and handle obstacles that appear suddenly in our path, will dictate the amount of success we are going to have in our life. Whether good or bad, no matter what has happened to us along the way, we have all made personal choices that have led us to where we are right now. None of us are exempt from problems, ridicule, and negativity from our peers. We are stressed out, over worked, exhausted, and our attitudes are in the gutter. So, what is next, how do we fix it and what things should we really concentrate on?

Lets discuss what I feel are the four major lifestyle choices that you must pay attention to; First in line is stress; then comes the importance of sleep. Third would be the significance of maintaining a positive mental attitude and lastly, but certainly not least is the importance of having a strong spiritual belief.

The first aspect of lifestyle choices that we are going to address has affected every single one of us, some more than others, and that is too much stress.

Stress

Stress is a huge topic for discussion; it is one of the main causes of our own self-destruction. We are bombarded with physical and emotional demands, hectic work schedules, increasing competitive pressures, prejudiced behaviors, marital problems, both spouses working, child behavior problems, finances, lack of direction/purpose in our careers and personal lives and these are just a few of the causes of stress.

There are two main types of stress I want to address, acute and chronic.

Acute Stress

Acute stress is a short-term response by the body's sympathetic nervous system. Basically it prepares us for fight or flight situations, and is usually short-term.

This type of stress may last a few days or a few weeks. During acute stress, our body releases many different hormones which cause our blood sugar levels to rise, and additional red blood cells to be released. Constriction of peripheral blood vessels also occurs, increasing blood pressure and pulse, and our digestion slows almost to a stop. An example of this would be if you suddenly noticed your wallet or purse where missing, your body now goes into a stage of acute stress. This is usually only temporary; it will last until you find your wallet/purse or until you rationally come up with some sort of a solution to the problem. In this example, your stress will gradually decrease over a short amount of time. The longer lasting and more dangerous type of stress is chronic stress.

Chronic Stress

Chronic stress is definitely the more serious of the two. It is constant and does not end. Our hectic, fast paced lifestyle continues to grind away at us, day by day adding increased pressures. This type of stress (chronic) is like a bag of water on each shoulder slowly filling more and more until we end up on our hands and knees with no more strength to keep moving. Our response to these demands is what brings on this so-called "chronic stress." Our body handles this stress in a variety of ways. Here is a list of some common stress related symptoms: irritability, anger, anxiety, depression, fatigue, tension headaches, stomachaches, hypertension, migraines, ulcers, heart attacks, or colitis. When our body gets really (chronic) stressed, it releases high amounts of a chemical called cortisol.

Cortisol is a natural hormone our body gives off in small amounts that are very beneficial. Cortisol is usually highest in our system in the early part of the day to get us up and moving and lowest at night. Good aspects of cortisol are:

- Inflammatory response
- Proper immune function
- Insulin release for blood sugar regulation
- Proper glucose metabolism
- Regulates blood pressure

Cortisol becomes a problem when increased stress occurs because our body releases greater quantities of cortisol. It can cause a variety of health problems. For example the most common are:

- Decreased immune function
- Increased weight gain
- Depression

Combat stress

There are many different ways to combat chronic stress. I want to list a few of the most common:

- Physical activity (any form)
- Meditation
- Massage
- Reading a book in a quite environment
- Watching your favorite movie
- Rest while listening to soft, quite music
- Yoga (stretching)
- Leisure activities, personally I enjoy golfing, fishing, and hiking.

Any one of these examples can be beneficial toward getting your mind in a more peaceful relaxed state. For more information about this topic, go to the web site, http://stress.about.com. or check out http://www.stressdirections.com.

Sleep

> "Without enough sleep, we all become tall two-year-olds."
>
> —JoJo Jensen

There is no question that most of us walk around all day half asleep. In today's lifestyle sleep depravation is very much on the rise. Most of us have become accustomed to surviving on coffee to get through each day. Lack of sleep has turned into a way of life. Most of us are fatigued so often that we think it is normal. Sleep depravation is actually the cause of many different problems. An article found at cnn.com about sleep depravation stated that scientists today are finding increased evidence that sleep deprivation has negative effects on appetite, strength of immune system, weight gain, risk of diabetes, and an increased risk to developing depression. More on this article at http://www.cnn.com. The National Sleep Foundation's 2005 sleep poll found that Americans on average are only getting 6.9 hours of sleep per night. 40% of people reported getting less than 7 hours of sleep per night. Only 49% reported actually getting a good night sleep. 62% of American's report having daytime sleepiness at least 3 times per week. Sleep related problems are estimated to cost Americans over $100 billion annually in lost productivity, medical expenses, sick leave, and property and environmental damage (National Sleep Foundation). The National Sleep Foundation's 2001 poll stated that about seven out of 10 Americans said that they experience frequent sleep problems, although most of them have not been diagnosed.

Melatonin and Sleep

Lack of sleep prevents the body from performing its natural duties, many of which occur during sleep. For example, there is a hormone released at night that is designed to help us relax and slow down. Our organs and our heart are slowed down in a relaxed state and our respiration (breathing) is slowed down. This hormone is called melatonin. It also acts as a powerful antioxidant to rid our bodies of toxins. When our bodies don't get the adequate sleep it requires then we don't use melatonin efficiently and we can suffer from premature aging, heart risks and cancer. An imbalance in melatonin levels has also been linked to depression. Hopefully by now we have a greater understanding on how important proper sleep is to a properly functioning, healthy body.

Positive Mental Attitude

> "I am still determined to be cheerful and happy, in whatever situation I may be; for I have also learned from experience that the greater part of our happiness or misery depends upon our dispositions, and not upon our circumstances."
>
> —Martha Washington

This is probably the hardest lifestyle attribute to achieve on a daily basis. We all know it is so much easier to go around in a bad mood, complaining about so and so, and just acting like we don't care. But what good are we doing? Are we helping ourselves? Are we helping anyone else? No, of course not! The one trait that can completely change the way we view ourselves, our jobs, and others is having a positive attitude. Here are a few statistics on the negative affects a poor attitude has lead to for many Americans. These stats are from the National Institute of Mental Health.

- In 2000, 29,350 people died by suicide in the U.S.
- Some 8 million to 14 million Americans suffer from depression each year.

We have all heard the saying "laughter is the best medicine." Did you know that laughing actually stimulates endorphins inside our bodies that promote healing which stimulate cellular activity? These natural endorphins also act as natural pain killers and produce an over all sense of well-being. At the University in California Dr. Lee Berk and Dr. Stanley Tan have been studying the effects of laughter on the immune system. Their published studies have shown that laughing lowers blood pressure, reduces stress hormones, increases muscle flexion, and boosts immune function by raising levels of infection-fighting T-cells, disease-fighting proteins called gamma-interferon and B-cells, which produce disease-destroying antibodies. This article is found at: http://www.holisticonline.com/Humor_Therapy/humor_therapy_benefits.htm.

I'll break this into a very simple and basic message, *Start Laughing*.

Stay out of the trap

There is no one given formula for having a positive mental attitude. It is a personal choice to rise above and separate yourself from the negative trap. We can all be negative and depressed but it takes a special person to have a positive attitude. You can completely change the way you feel about life by changing your attitude. People are drawn to this attribute. How many great leaders do you know that were or are depressed and negative people? I can't think of anyone. Success comes from perseverance and perseverance is just a fifty-cent word for positive mental attitude. You will find a more fulfilling life, an increase of personal achievements, and you will see more doors opening for you. Once you have made your choice and transformed your attitude, stay out of the negative trap. Once you have fallen in, it is very hard to get back out!

Guidance, Direction, and Purpose

> "Be strong and have great courage. Be not afraid, neither be though dismayed for the Lord they God is with you where ever you go"
>
> —Joshua 1–9

What is life without purpose? What is life without a foundation? What is life without basic principles to follow? NOTHING! We all need to have something that we follow and believe.

Joshua 1–9 is my favorite quote in the Bible. I have turned to this quote many times in my life for strength and encouragement. I even had this on the front of one of my binders when I was in college. However, without believing that it was true, what purpose or good would it serve? This section of the book is not intended to shove my personal beliefs onto any of you. Dr. Kosinski and I wanted to add this simply to show the importance of having a strong foundation to live by with guidelines to follow. I do know what has worked for my family, my wife and myself. I will write briefly from personal experience but, first let's talk about an actual research study that has proven real positive benefits of having spiritual faith.

Research provided by Christopher G. Ellison, PhD, of the University of Texas, Austin, and Jeffrey S. Levin, PhD, of the National Institute of Healthcare Research, Rockville, MD makes a compelling case that religion plays a big part associated with better overall health.

- Healthy Behavior. Religious involvement may discourage behavior that increases health risks, such as tobacco and alcohol consumption, or it may encourage other positive lifestyle choices.
- Social Support. People who regularly attend religious services appear to have larger and denser social networks to provide emotional support and other forms of assistance than less frequent attendees.
- Self Esteem. Religious involvement may promote feelings of self-worth and confidence in the ability to control one's own affairs and destiny.

- Coping Skills. Prayer, meditation and other religious activities may help people deal with stressful events and conditions.
- Positive Emotions. Religious activities may also lead to positive emotions, which have been shown to influence immune functions and other physiological factors that influence health. More on this article at: http://www.sciencedaily.com/releases/1998/10/981030081243.htm

The main reason I am the person that I am today and in the position that I am in is because of my personal faith. The best thing my parents did for me growing up was instilling the principles of the Bible in me. All my strength, happiness, and personal success has been led and guided by my faith and belief in God. You must have a strong foundation and guidelines in your life to follow or you're just another leaf on the branch waiting for your time to fall off the tree and slowly wilt away. I cannot stress enough the importance of this lifestyle aspect. Seek out your spiritual questions today; don't wait for tomorrow. Time isn't something any one of us can afford to waste.

Good luck my friends on your new journey to a life you have only seen in your dreams. You can now own this dream life, and turn your life circumstances into new and positive opportunities. Dr. Kosinski and I wish you well on your new path and we are very excited to be a part of your life transformation. We leave you with the quote that was the inspiration for this book!

"A committed heart does not wait for conditions to be exactly right. Why? Because conditions are never exactly right. Indecision limits the Almighty and His ability to perform miracles in your life. He has put the vision in you—proceed! To wait, to wonder, to doubt, to be indecisive is to disobey God."

—Andy Andrews

Appendix A
Websites

Chiropractic

www.icpa4kids.org

www.yourspine.com

www.chiroweb.com

www.becomehealthynow.com

www.gonstead.com

Lifestyle

http://stress.about.com

http://www.stressdirections.com

http://www.cnn.com

http://www.holisticonline.com/Humor_Therapy/humor_therapy_benefits.htm.

http://www.sciencedaily.com/releases/1998/10/981030081243.htm

Exercise

http://news.bbc.co.uk/1/hi/health/4778274.stm.

http://exercise.about.com.

http://www2.gsu.edu/~wwwfit/strength.html

Diet

http://www.healthdangers.com/drugs/MSG/index.htm

http://www.msgtruth.org/related.htm

http://www.holisticmed.com/aspartame/summary.html.

http://splendaexposed.com.

http://stevia.com.

http://www.xylitol.org

http://www.thebodybygod.com/

http://www.vegsoc.org/.

http://www.mercola.com/nutritionplan/juicing.htm.

http://www.powerjuicer.com

http://www.healingdaily.com/juicing-for-health/juicing-recipes.htm.

http://www.bodyforlife.com.

Appendix B

The Top 11 Questions About Chiropractic

1. Q: What is Chiropractic?

A: Chiropractic is based on the scientific fact that your body is a self-regulating, self-healing organism controlled by the brain, spinal cord and nerves. The 24 bones of the spine, or vertebrae, surround and protect the spinal cord. When misaligned, or subluxated, the vertebrae can interfere with the nervous system, causing pain and dysfunction.

As chiropractors, our objective is to analyze the spine, locate and correct these vertebral subluxations. The chiropractic method of correction is by specific adjustments of the spinal bones (vertebrae), which are intended to correct vertebral subluxations over time, thereby allowing the innate (inborn) healing abilities of the body to work at maximum efficiency.

2. Q: What is a vertebral subluxation?

A: Before you learn what a vertebral subluxation is, you must first know how the body works. According to "Gray's Anatomy" (renowned medical text), the purpose of the brain and nervous system is to control and coordinate the function of all organs, glands and tissues in the body.

The brain directs and controls all organ function, muscles, and joint movement by sending messages or impulses along the nerves to the various parts of the body and then back again. Any interference in this communication results in reduced organ function, movement, and health.

A *vertebral subluxation* is a condition that causes interference with the nerve communication system.

1. A *vertebral subluxation* is a structural misalignment of spinal bones (vertebrae) of the spine.
2. A *vertebral subluxation*, (bone misalignments) can cause the opening from which the nerves exit to become narrowed.
3. A narrow opening may compress (impinge, choke) the nerve.
4. The nerve may become damaged, and affects body function and your health.

3. **Q: What causes vertebral subluxations?**

A: The causes of vertebral subluxation are the obvious things such as: sports injuries, motor vehicle accidents, slips and falls ... etc. Less obvious, and far more common, vertebral subluxations can be caused by the cumulative effects of our bad habits: bad posture, poor diet, unhealthy sleeping positions and especially—poor ergonomics in the work place. Research from Pediatric and Developmental Chiropractic is showing that the most common first spinal trauma, and therefore the first cause of vertebral subluxation, is the birth process and the delivery itself.

4. Q: Do you feel vertebral Subluxations

A: A vertebral subluxation is a degenerative problem. Therefore it starts silently and evolves into a weakness that we may aggravate or "tweak". This leads to increased swelling and nerve pressure until a thresh hold of tolerance is crossed and we experience some type of symptom, or warning signal from the body. These body signals tend to occur well into the development of this problem. Symptoms of nerve pressure and dysfunction may include weakness, restlessness, tingling or numbness, organ dysfunction, asthma, allergies, stomach problems, bowel problems, ear or sinus problems and eventually some type of pain syndrome or crisis. Symptoms typically occur at the end of a problem, not at the beginning. As with teeth, cholesterol, and heart problems, it is never wise to wait for the symptoms associated with crisis. Have your spine and nerve system checked proactively.

5. Q: What is a chiropractic adjustment?

A: A chiropractic adjustment is a carefully directed and controlled pressure applied to a spinal joint that is subluxated, or not moving properly. The chiropractic adjustment removes vertebral subluxations and restores motion to the joints, helping the bones of the spine gradually return to a more normal position and motion. With improved position and motion, there is decreased interference with the nervous system, increased communication within the body, and improved overall balance.

After many years of training, a chiropractor is an expert at using the correct amount of force in the correct direction. Some adjustments may require a quick movement, and others involve slow and constant pressure. After a thorough examination, we determine which technique will work best for you.

6. **Q: Does it hurt to get adjusted?**

A: Adjustments do NOT hurt. The doctor has learned how and where to adjust properly and pain-free. On the other hand, you should NEVER try to "adjust" yourself as you may cause more pain or increase the damage that has occurred.

7. **Q: What causes the sound during an adjustment?**

A: Actually, adjustments do not always produce a sound. Often, however, adjustments do create the sound of a spinal "release," or "popping" sound. The sound is caused by gas rushing in to fill the partial vacuum created when the joints are slightly separated. This sound is painless and totally harmless.

8. **Q: Why can't I just get adjusted once?**

A: Correcting the problem subluxation requires a series of specific, gentle adjustments to the spine in order to "train" the nerve system and structures back toward a healthier position and function. The body's tissues have a "memory". Because vertebral subluxations typically develop and worsen over time, this unhealthy "memory" must now be "reprogrammed" in order to get a positive and lasting result. This correction process is much like wearing braces on teeth. The correction in this case however results in a healthier spine and nerve system, not just a prettier smile.

9. **Q: Do I have to get adjusted forever?**

A: Only as long as you want the benefits. Just as with working-out, regardless of an individual's fitness level, they must continue to put in the time and effort training to maintain and/or increase their fitness level. If at any time they quit working-out, they simply lose what they've gained over time. The same is true with chiropractic, and anything in our lives of value for that matter. The benefits of chiropractic care are yours as long as it is part of your life.

10. **Q: Is Chiropractic Safe.**

A: Records from insurance and court cases have constantly shown that chiropractic is the safest portal of entry health care available to the public today. Although no healthcare procedures are 100% safe, chiropractic stands on its record of safety and effectiveness unmatched in healthcare. To learn more about the safety record of chiropractic please visit the website Chiropractic Is Safe at www.chiropracticissafe.org

11. **Q: How much education do Doctors of Chiropractic need?**

A: After completing their undergraduate education, chiropractors receive an additional four years of post-graduate education and a two-year internship to become a Doctor of Chiropractic. Their education curriculum is similar to medical school and there is special emphasis on anatomy, physiology, neurology, biomechanics, nutrition, X-ray, and spinal adjusting techniques. To become a licensed chiropractor, he or she must pass a demanding four-part National Board Examination and then a State Board examination for the state in which they wish to practice. A chiropractor's education never stops, as yearly continuing education is required for license renewal.

About The Authors

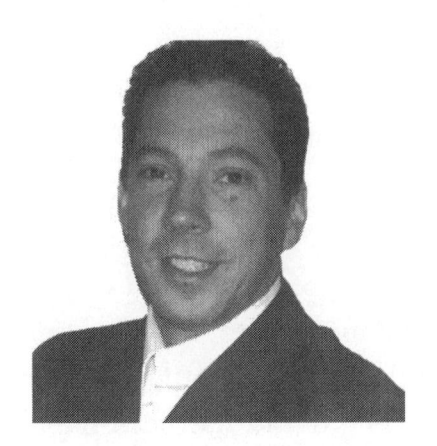

John Kosinski, BS, DC

Dr. John Kosinski was born and raised in Cambridge, Ma. He received his Bachelor of Science degree from Northeastern University in Boston, and later was the owner of a successful janitorial company in Woburn, MA. John then went on to receive his Doctor of Chiropractic degree from Sherman College of Straight Chiropractic. He is an avid weekend athlete, playing ice hockey and traveling the country with his fast pitch softball team. John believes that the body is the most amazing, self healing; self regulating creation on the planet. His goal is to reach as many people as he can with the message that "you can live to be 100 but feel like you're 20", if you are willing to put in a little bit of effort. John Currently resides in Manchester, NH with his wife Dr. April Kosinski and they are both in private practice with Dr. Joshua Ebert.

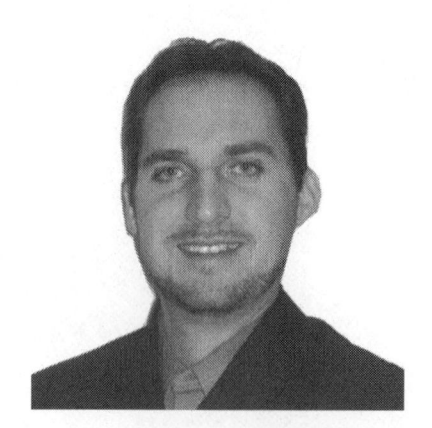

Joshua Ebert, BS, DC

Dr. Joshua Ebert grew up on the west coast. His father was in the air force so they moved around a lot until his late teenage years where he and his family settled in Eastern Washington. Dr. Ebert is 29 years old and has been happily married to his wife Keri for the past 6 years. Their recent family addition is a puppy named Kloey. Since high school he has always had a passion for health and nutrition. Dr. Ebert definitely lives what he preaches. He loves fitness and weight training, follows a regular healthy eating program and is not only a Chiropractor, but is also a regular patient. Dr. Ebert chose chiropractic as a career because he felt it was a perfect balance of natural health and wellness. His pursuit of Chiropractic led him to receive both a Bachelor of Science and Doctor of Chiropractic degrees. His desire is to educate as many people as possible about the true path towards achieving optimal health.

978-0-595-43988-1
0-595-43988-8

Printed in Great Britain
by Amazon.co.uk, Ltd.,
Marston Gate.